Fibromyalgia
For
Families and Friends

What You Need to Know to Support Your Loved One with Fibromyalgia

Janet L Black, RN, FNP, MSN, MPH

Peaceful Heart Press
Candler, North Carolina

Copyright 2014 by Janet L Black and Peaceful Heart Press

All rights reserved. No part of this manuscript may be reproduced, stored in a retrieval system or transmitted in any form or by any means, electronic, mechanical, photocopying, recording or otherwise without the written permission of the author.

Disclaimer: While the author and publisher have used their best efforts in preparing this book, they make no representations or warranties with respect to the accuracy or completeness of the contents of this book. The advice and strategies contained herein shall not be construed as medical, psychiatric or psychological advice. You should consult with a professional where appropriate. Neither the publisher nor the author shall be held liable for any loss or damages.

Other books by Janet L Black:

The Road to Healing: A Guide to Recovering from Sexual Abuse

Lose Weight without Hunger: The Secret to Permanent Weight Loss

Foreword

I would like to thank all my friends with fibromyalgia, who in sharing their stories of encounters with other people who just "didn't get it" made me aware of the need for a simple, concise explanation that we could give to our families, or friends and our doctors to help them understand us. It has occurred to me as I have written this book that even my family, who haven't taken any of the blatantly unsupportive positions that I have heard of from others, probably don't fully understand what it is like to have this condition.

This book is dedicated to my fibromyalgia support group who have become like family and taught me more than my medical training did about this condition and how to live with it.

I would like to thank my husband for his unswerving support during all of our years together. I suspect that I had fibromyalgia before meeting him but was unaware of it as I did not develop significant symptoms until later. Many of my friends have not been as fortunate and some have been abandoned by people who did not want to continue a relationship with someone who had a chronic illness.

I hope that this little book will enlighten my readers and help them to have more fulfilling relationships with the people around them with fibromyalgia. Maybe we will stop hearing those dreaded words, "but you don't look sick".

Table of Contents

Fibromyalgia is an Invisible Illness

Chronic Pain

Energy and Sleep

Fibro-fog

Grieving and Depression

Other Symptoms and Associated Conditions

A Day in the Life

How You Can Support Us

Fibromyalgia is an Invisible Illness

When you see someone who is in a wheelchair or using a cane, you can tell they have something wrong and you don't question it when they pull into a handicapped parking space. There are a lot of other handicapped people with disabilities that you can't see but that are just as real. People with fibromyalgia don't look sick. When you see us, we are probably well-groomed, may look happy and look just like everyone else. Of course, you may only see us on our good days. Unless you live with us, you don't see us on the days that it is an effort to even get out of bed and we don't even get dressed, far less go anywhere. Even if you do live with us, it can be difficult to understand why sometimes we seem normal and other days we don't want to do anything. There are times when we may be irritable and whine about our pain but most of the time, we try to hide it and act as normal as we can. This does not mean that we feel normal. We can smile and laugh even when we are in pain. We are used to hurting; it is our "normal". It is hard to explain fibromyalgia to someone who doesn't have it but so many of my fibro friends have told me about family and friends that just don't "get it" that I decided I should write a book to help explain it to "normal people". I have been blessed to have family and friends that are supportive but I'm sure that they don't really understand just what it is like to live with this every day for years and what it does to your life. This book describes what it is like although it might be a little different for each person.

I should probably give you a little information on my background. I have fibromyalgia. It often starts after some kind of trauma and cervical strain is a common one. I think it may have started for me with a car accident where I was hit from behind and had whiplash, otherwise known as cervical strain. I think I lost consciousness briefly and felt confused afterward. I knew I should do something after the accident but couldn't remember what. I took down driver's license information from the guy who hit me and drove home. When I got home, my husband noticed that the frame of the car was bent and he took me to the police station to report the accident and then took me to get medical care. Since the person who hit me didn't have a valid license or insurance, it is no wonder that he didn't remind me that we should call the police. Not only did my neck hurt but I developed a headache that lasted for about three months and when I went for physical therapy, the therapist discovered that I was balancing with my eyes. If I closed my eyes, I would lose my balance. She worked with me on balance. Eventually the headaches stopped and I got better.

Within a few years of that time, I went back to school to become a family nurse practitioner. When I studied fibromyalgia, I learned about the tender points used to diagnose it and I had all 18 of them. I wasn't aware of having any other symptoms at that time. One of the physician preceptors I worked with, told me that he thought fibromyalgia was not real but just a condition that people used to get disability. I was inclined to agree since he was the expert and I had the tender points but didn't have it (that I knew of).

Fast forward a couple years and I was at the doctor's office complaining about fatigue. I just didn't have any energy. I tried an antidepressant but it did nothing to help. Then I was back, complaining about pain in my neck and shoulders all of the time. Naproxen was prescribed and while it usually works really well on me for muscle strains, it had no effect. I began having pain in other areas as well and then started having difficulty sleeping. I fell three times in three months and the third time, sprained my ankle quite badly. I began putting all of these things together, particularly the pain and sleep difficulties and wondered if this could be fibromyalgia. I had been working and treating patients with it before this time and as a result, I began to see it as a real condition. After I self-diagnosed it as fibromyalgia, I saw my primary care provider and got a referral to a rheumatologist since she didn't feel comfortable making the diagnosis. One of my co-workers told me that I didn't have it and that it wasn't real. The rheumatologist diagnosed me as having fibromyalgia.

I was doing lots of reading and learning all I could. I joined an on-line support group of fibromyalgia sufferers and they told me about symptoms I wasn't aware of being part of the disease but that I had. They contributed more to my education about fibromyalgia than the professional literature because they were in the trenches, having to deal with this condition everyday of their lives. They are a great group and we have all become very close friends who support each other through all the different things that we and our families have happen. It really helps to have other people who understand what we are going through.

It is still not known what causes fibromyalgia although it has been linked to injuries, infections and post-traumatic stress disorder. What is known is that it is a central nervous system disorder where the person feels pain more intensely. It affects more women than it does men. It is not psychological; it is physical. People sometimes say it is just in our heads. Well, our brains, a part of the central nervous system, are in our heads so in that respect they are correct but it is not a mental condition or our imagination. Are people with fibromyalgia depressed? Wouldn't you be if you had to live with chronic pain, a lack of energy, difficulty sleeping etc.? We have had to suffer so many losses of things we can no longer do that it would be a miracle if we didn't feel depressed sometimes. That doesn't mean that it results from depression or is a psychological problem. While stress can make it worse, reducing stress will not cure it and in fact, there is no known cure. Anyone who claims to have cured it probably didn't have it in the first place. It is called a syndrome rather than a disease because of the fact that the cause and much of how it produces effects on the body, are not understood yet.

While pain is a huge problem for us, it is not only pain. People with fibromyalgia are more sensitive to noise, bright lights, odors and pressure. Put me in a place with flashing lights and noise such as an arcade or certain restaurants that cater to children and I want to leave immediately. If I want to move furniture, I will probably want to use hot pads on my hands to help relieve the pain that the pressure of lifting something heavy causes. I use a rubber thing to open jars because gripping them hard enough to open them, hurts otherwise. It isn't a lack of strength but a matter of the pressure on my hands. And forget kneeling because that is way too painful. Even sitting can hurt. There are lots of little adjustments that we make and things we know to avoid as we learn to live with this condition.

It also affects our brain so that we have lapses in memory and problems with coordination and balance. I will talk more about the memory issues in the chapter on fibro fog. I don't like stairs and will always use a railing and have a cane to use if I am on uneven ground to help prevent falls. My balance got worse with the onset of other fibromyalgia symptoms. By the time I realize I am falling, it is too late to stop myself. I am very cautious because I know what is risky for me and I want to avoid injury.

Fibromyalgia is diagnosed by the presence of widespread pain (in upper and lower body and on both sides) that has lasted over three months, fatigue, an absence of other causes for the symptoms (usually by means of blood tests that come back normal) and by the presence of tender points. For diagnosis, at least 11 of the 18 tender points should be painful when pressure is put on them. Some people go to many different doctors for years before they are diagnosed. It only took me a year and a half because I was a healthcare professional and figured it out myself.

One of the things that baffles our friends is that sometimes we seem to be fine and at other times we "flare" and wind up cancelling plans. I make plans on the basis that I expect to be okay. Usually I am. If we cancel plans, it isn't you and it isn't anything we can predict. Doing too much and having more stress can send us into a "flare" so we try not to plan too much and try to keep our stress levels low. But it is not a guarantee. I can rest up so I will be in good shape to do something and still not be up to doing it. Sometimes, the things I don't do are things I actually want very much to do and I may be more disappointed than you are if I have to cancel. I will push myself to do as much as I can but sometimes I know that pushing any more will have consequences and I need to rest and relax for a while. When you have fibromyalgia, you have to learn to listen to your body.

The experts say that fibromyalgia is not a progressive disease but I have watched friends get worse over time. After seeing my own health gradually get worse, I turned to alternative medicine and have seen some improvement. I also use diet and exercise to attempt to stay as healthy as possible. When I was first diagnosed, the rheumatologist told me to join a gym or I would be in a wheelchair within a year. I am grateful that she was wrong because I never joined a gym and I'm still walking around on my own but I do exercise. Research indicates that exercise benefits those with fibromyalgia but one has to use caution because too much can definitely lead to a flare. It is a delicate balance to try to be as active as we can, without overdoing it. You might not think we are doing much but we know we have to be cautious.

Fibromyalgia won't kill us but it certainly affects the quality of our lives. We appreciate the family and friends who are willing to listen to us, try to understand, stick by us and support us. Thank you for reading this book!

Chronic Pain

The pain of fibromyalgia is what we call neuropathic pain. This means that it is nerve pain similar to the pain of diabetic peripheral neuropathy or shingles. Because it is nerve pain, the same kinds of medication are used to treat it. It is different than the kind of pain you have with an injury or from arthritis (which is inflammatory pain) and so different kinds of medication that work on the central nervous system are more effective than medications for inflammatory pain. So acetaminophen will work better than naproxen or ibuprofen (although acetaminophen is rarely going to be strong enough to have a significant effect).

When people ask me to describe what the pain is like, I ask them if they have ever signed up at a gym after not exercising and then gone crazy using all the weight machines at the highest weight they can plus doing aerobics for an hour. Then I ask them to remember how they felt the next couple of days when every muscle in their body ached, even the bottoms of their feet, so that they didn't want to move. Imagine feeling like that every day, all day. With an overuse type of pain, holding still helps. For fibromyalgia pain, it doesn't. Of course, some days are better and some are worse (with the pain being more like recovering from surgery) but that gives people a little bit of an idea of what it is like to live with chronic pain that is never really gone. It may hurt more in different places on different days. Ever had shingles? Everyone talks about how incredibly painful they are. I have had them and I didn't even take pain meds for them. I feel like that all the time and have just learned to live with it. I have some pain medications on hand in case I have a flare and try not to take them. I do take supplements that help by increasing serotonin and by reducing nerve reactivity.

Besides the deep aching, the pain can also be sharp, burning or tingly and can be so severe as to be incapacitating. There can be sensitivity to touch and pressure. The sensitivity to pressure can feel like your entire body is bruised. Everyone is different and pain is a subjective experience so what I experience may not be the same as someone else. I suspect I had a fairly high pain tolerance to begin with so tolerate the pain from fibromyalgia better than some others do.

Many people take narcotic medications to cope with the pain so that they are able to do things that they couldn't do otherwise. Some doctors don't believe that people with a chronic condition like fibromyalgia should take narcotic medications because it is possible to build tolerance to them over time. That means that as your body gets used to them, they become less effective so that it takes more medication to achieve the same level of pain relief. Tolerance is not the same thing as addiction where a person craves the drug to get high. Tolerance is a normal response of the body but it makes it difficult to treat chronic pain because the patient may eventually want more of the medication to get the same amount of relief. When someone is dying of cancer, the doctors will just increase the dose and not worry about it but if someone is going to need pain relief for another 30, 40 or 50 years, tolerance can be a problem. It is why I don't take narcotics except on rare occasions with a severe flare and I encourage others not to start them on a regular basis if possible. But when the pain gets severe and the person is already taking everything nonnarcotic available to prevent it, then there is no other good option.

That being said, I hear stories constantly about doctors who stop narcotics, don't refill them on time and basically allow patients to suffer. Once a person is on narcotic medication, stopping it abruptly causes the person to have worse pain than they would have if they had never taken any because they have the pain of withdrawal on top of what pain they would have had anyway. Far too often, patients with chronic pain get labeled as "drug seeking" which is a nice way of saying "addict". Of course, we are drug seeking. We want the pain to stop and failing that, at least be reduced to a manageable level. That doesn't mean we are addicts. Emergency rooms are especially notorious for treating patients with fibromyalgia badly and most of us try to avoid them when possible. The medical journals actually contribute to some of this by saying that fibromyalgia should not be treated with narcotics and that they are not that effective for our pain. They are effective and sometimes the pain is so severe that nothing else works. The same doctor who would happily prescribe narcotics for other conditions may balk at treating fibromyalgia pain.

Years ago, I went to my primary care doctor and requested a prescription for tramadol. This is a medication that is not classified as a narcotic although it works like a mild narcotic. I didn't want to take it every day. I wanted it on hand just in case I needed it. I had to beg and plead to talk my doctor into 25 tablets which lasted me for a few years! I need to have something on hand for those times when I am flaring enough to need it. It is sort of a security blanket. When you flare, you need something right then and don't want to have to go to an urgent care or emergency room where they are very suspicious of people wanting narcotics for chronic pain. It is much better to get something in a regular physician's office where you hope you have built a relationship of trust. Most people with fibromyalgia are open to trying anything that might work and want to use the lowest dose of narcotics they can get by on and still function. Not all medications work on all people. Some don't relieve the pain and some have side effects that are so awful, that we cannot tolerate them. We have learned how different medications affect us and really need our healthcare providers to work with us to help us get adequate pain relief.

Doctors (or other healthcare providers who prescribe drugs such as nurse practitioners and physician assistants) may be concerned about prescribing narcotics to a chronic pain patient because of the DEA (Drug Enforcement Agency), the federal agency which monitors the use of controlled substances or state agencies that function in a similar manner. Treatment with narcotics has to be documented properly so the patient should be seen monthly and be reporting the level of pain before and after taking medication and what things they are able to do as a result of pain relief. Not all primary care providers are prepared to do this so the patient may have to go to a pain specialist. Hopefully, the person you know who suffers from fibromyalgia has found a good, reliable provider who listens, documents carefully, works with the patient and prescribes what is needed. Sometimes, it takes a bit of effort to find a good provider who understands our condition. If we seem like we "doctor shop", we are just trying to find someone who listens, believes us and will work with us to develop an effective treatment plan.

Despite all the information in the professional literature showing that fibromyalgia is real, there are still some providers who don't believe this. I have heard plenty of horror stories from friends about poor treatment from doctors.

The worst case was where one of my friends went to see a physician regarding a gastrointestinal issue. He challenged her diagnosis of fibromyalgia and decided that she was bi-polar, although he had no expertise in mental health. She had, in fact, been seen by mental health professionals who determined that she had no mental illness. Despite this, he had her involuntarily hospitalized as being suicidal in a mental health institution where she was given medication she was allergic to and traumatized. Her husband was not even told where she was and she was held longer than the legally allowed amount of time without any legal representation. This is an extreme case but I have heard from many people with fibromyalgia tell about instances where they were treated with disrespect and disdain because of their diagnosis and need for pain relief. Some doctors will refuse to take patients who have fibromyalgia. I have attempted to refer patients to a rheumatologist only to be told that I could refer someone with any other diagnosis except fibromyalgia. It can be really difficult for us to find a good doctor.

Families and friends can worry about addiction when someone they care about is taking narcotics. We have all heard stories of someone who got "hooked" on prescription pain pills but with most chronic pain patients, this does not happen. Most of the patients I have run into who had an addiction problem with prescription narcotics had some sort of acute pain and when they got better, they liked the effect of the narcotics and wanted to keep taking them. Since the pain was gone, they were taking them for the high they got and to prevent withdrawal symptoms. This is very different from taking them to relieve pain. Your loved one is not going to suddenly turn into a drug addict because they need narcotic pain medication to function. If they are taking their medication as prescribed, then don't worry about it. It is a matter for the doctor/NP/PA and the patient.

Energy and Sleep

One of the other classic symptoms of fibromyalgia is fatigue or a lack of energy. Even after a good night's sleep, a person with fibromyalgia may feel so tired that he or she can barely drag out of bed. This fatigue can last all day or it can improve. It can get worse later in the day. In general, I find that it is hard to get going in the morning and I usually don't have a lot of energy in the evening so afternoons are my best time. I used to be a morning person, cheerfully bouncing out of bed each day. This was somewhat annoying to my husband who was not a morning person but he no longer has to be concerned; my excessive morning cheerfulness has been tempered by feeling stiff and achy and with less energy.

One of the best descriptions I have read of how it is to live with a chronic illness that affects energy levels was written by Christine Miserandino, who has the website www.butyoudon'tlooksick.com and who developed The Spoon Theory. I urge you to read it. She was trying to explain to a friend what it felt like to have lupus and was in a restaurant at the time. She gathered up a handful of spoons, handed them to her friend and explained to her friend that the spoons each represented a unit of energy. Each thing that she did used energy so she started out with a number of spoons and as she got up, showered, dressed, fixed breakfast etc., each one of those activities took away a spoon. Each day, a person with a chronic illness must make a choice with the limited number of spoons, or units of energy, about what they are going to spend them on. Normal people have unlimited choices of what they can spend their time doing while we have to think about the effects of everything we do and whether we will have the energy to do what we want. To add to that, we don't even know how many "spoons" we have for the day. We can do a few things and then run out of energy.

I often think of all kinds of plans regarding what I would like to do but I have to prioritize because chances are, I'm not going to be able to do all of them. I try to choose the activities that are most important to me. I accept that sometimes things are not going to get done. Actually, even with choosing a limited number of things, I often don't get everything done since I still want to think I can function like a normal person and have unrealistic expectations. So, if I fix a great dinner, I might not wash the dishes until the next day. By evening, I am often running out of energy. I have had days where I don't even get dressed but put my energy into writing instead. I try not to schedule too many things on the same day. But sometimes, I don't have control of the schedule and there are several things I want to go to on the same day. I try to rest ahead of time and push myself to do them all. Sometimes it works and sometimes it doesn't. Things like housework, which I hate doing anyway, can get pushed back until I have to do it or I happen to have a high energy day.

One of the things that helps us is pacing. Not the walking back and forth kind but the taking of frequent rest breaks and not pushing ourselves excessively. We have all learned the consequences of not pacing ourselves. If we push ourselves to do too much, the next morning, we feel like we have been run over by a truck. This experience of more pain and less energy is what we call a "flare" and trying to do too much can bring one on. So, if I am helping you do something and I decide to go sit down for five or ten minutes and rest, this is healthy behavior on my part. I am taking care of myself and will be able to do more in the long run than if I didn't take those rest breaks. It also means not trying to do too much on one day but breaking up tasks or activities and spreading them out over a few days.

Another one of our problems is disturbances in sleep. We don't tend to sleep well and when we are in pain, it is worse. We need comfortable beds, lots of pillows and a room that is not too hot or cold (we are sensitive to temperature). Foam and extra pillows can help prevent too much pressure on any one area of the body. I have a four inch pad of memory foam on top of my mattress and sleep with three pillows. This can be a concern when we sleep away from home because in an uncomfortable, hard bed, we could be awake all night.

While no one is sure what causes sleep problems for people with fibromyalgia, one theory is that we have abnormal brain chemicals. Research using brain wave studies has found that instead of normal sleep cycles which go through five levels of sleep from light sleep to deep sleep, we don't get the deep sleep where the body restores and refreshes itself. It is during these stages of sleep that the body releases chemicals such as growth hormone that help with tissue repair. The lack of deep sleep may play a role in cognitive problems such as fibro fog since these stages of sleep are necessary to process memories. We may have alterations in levels of some neurotransmitters that send messages in the brain and in hormones such as cortisol which affect our ability to sleep and could also worsen pain. This could also be one factor in the fatigue or lack of energy we experience.

I don't advise anyone to use sleeping pills to improve sleep as they are habit forming. I personally take a muscle relaxer. This was the first medication I took for fibromyalgia, started by the rheumatologist. It works on the central nervous system, not the muscles and does help me to sleep. I am still on the same dose of one tablet at bedtime. I also take melatonin and gamma amino butyric acid (GABA), natural substances found in the brain to help induce sleep and calm the nervous system. I generally sleep very well using these. This is not to say that I have no fatigue but I think it would be far worse if I were not taking them. I have seen some improvement in memory and I have less pain since adding the GABA. It is related to **gaba**pentin (Neurontin) and pre**gaba**lin (Lyrica) but without the side effects or high prescription drug price. I also find that avoiding the computer screen and instead, doing some reading before bed helps with sleep. Avoiding stimulants such as caffeine and exercise in the evening also helps with relaxation and sleep.

Fibro-fog

One of the reasons that I can't work at a regular job is fibro-fog. This is a condition where my brain simply doesn't work correctly. Most of the time I am fine but in my foggy moments, I can't remember words, especially names of things. Sometimes, I say the wrong word. I don't remember what I am supposed to do that day or where I put things. I walk into a room and don't know why I am there. Usually I have a great memory but have had times when I couldn't remember my Social Security number or similar basic information. I may have difficulty concentrating. I don't learn as easily as I used to because I may not remember what I learned yesterday.

Many of us are not as comfortable in social settings because of our intermittently foggy brains. If you ask me something and get a "deer in the headlights" blank stare, it is because I am struggling to find information that I just can't access right then. You know the game "Taboo" where you have to get someone to guess a word without using it or certain other words? You have to describe it and hope the person can guess. Well, I often feel like I am playing that game. It is a good thing that my husband is good at guessing. As you can imagine, this isn't something I want to do with strangers. It is no wonder that I like to communicate via email so I have time to think about what I want to say. When I am going to do any public speaking, I have the speech written out so I can read it if my mind goes blank.

You can probably imagine how difficult it would be to provide health care to someone when you recognize their condition but can't remember what it is called or the name of the medication used to treat it. That means you can't simply look it up. Sometimes, by spending more time with the patient, it would come to me but I couldn't count on that. I might also forget to ask some questions or do some part of an exam. One place where I worked was slow about filing lab and x-ray results so I might see the patient after signing off on them but before they were in the chart. One day, I could tell the patient the exact number of an abnormal lab result and another day, I couldn't even remember that they had the test. Between the fibro-fog, the pain and the lack of energy, I eventually had to give up. Even trying to reduce stress and work part-time didn't work. I was fortunate to get disability on my first application without having to appeal.

As an author, I don't make much money but can work when I'm feeling good, on my own schedule. I don't have to do anything on the days when I have no energy or can't concentrate. If I don't remember something, I can look it up or come back to it later. It does result in some stress but nothing like trying to provide healthcare and be afraid of making an error that could affect a patient. I do have frustration in working with computer programs because I can't remember how I did something the last time I did it. I have to figure things out several times and even then, may forget how to do something. Everything seems harder with fibromyalgia but I want to do what I can. It is important to me to feel like I am doing something productive, even with my limitations. I hear this from my friends with fibromyalgia too. We want to do things and be productive and are frustrated when we can't. For me, writing allows me to use my background and education to help others and that makes me feel like I am contributing to society

Grieving and Depression

Having fibromyalgia means losing many of the good things in our lives. Some of us have lost spouses, friends, jobs and the ability to do things that brought us pleasure in addition to our health. Losing these things causes us to be in a state of grief and leads to feeling depressed.

Many of us have had to give up careers because of our fibromyalgia. If you think we are lucky because we "don't have to work", I want you to think about the last few times you had to stay home from work because you were sick. If someone offered you the opportunity to stay home every day at 25% of your normal salary but that you had to be sick all the time, what would you say? Does it sound like a good trade to you? It sure doesn't to me.

For many of us, fibromyalgia has meant a descent into poverty and a series of losses related to that. Imagine what happens when you lose your job. Unemployment doesn't pay that well and you can't find another job easily because of your limitations. You might not be able to pay your mortgage and lose your home, including whatever equity you might have built up over the years. You can't pay other bills and your credit rating plunges. This makes it hard for you to buy anything else using credit. Getting Social Security Disability is a slow process and you may have to appeal several times before you get it. Even if you get it, you won't get Medicare to cover your health expenses for two years. Since you lost your health insurance along with your job and you are sick, you are paying out of pocket for your medical expenses. If you had any savings, you have used them up during this time.

Many people on disability don't like anyone to know that they are getting it because when you don't look sick, people think you are somehow scamming the system and they tend to be prejudiced against you. Let me tell you, getting disability is not easy and you don't get it if you aren't actually disabled. Only 40% of those who apply are ever approved. It is called Social Security Disability Insurance because that is what it is. It is insurance that you pay into while you are working so that it covers you in the event that you become disabled. It is deducted from your paycheck. The other type of Social Security Disability is for those who are poor and too disabled to be able to work. You cannot have any savings or other valuable assets. Neither of these programs are going to give you lots of money. They are programs we use because we cannot work, not because we don't want to work.

I was depressed when I got the notice that I qualified for SSDI because although I needed the money, it was a confirmation that I really was in bad enough shape to qualify. I really wanted to be healthy. Losing your health permanently is enough to make anyone feel depressed.

Even those who can continue to work, which I did for ten years after I started having symptoms, usually are grieving for something that they have had to give up. Just having to endure the pain and lack of energy is difficult and after working all day, there is probably no energy left for going out or doing anything that is fun. I had to hire someone to come in and clean house because I couldn't. While giving up housework was certainly no loss, the fact that I was unable to do it was. I spent that ten years trying to hide my symptoms from employers so that I could continue to work. I had planned to work for another ten years. Fibromyalgia puts an end to a lot of future plans.

It is not unusual for spouses and friends to abandon us as we become more disabled because we can't go do fun things with them anymore. We cancel plans at the last minute. We go out but then want to go home early because we are fatigued. Even fun activities can wear us out. Some spouses are verbally abusive because they just don't understand us. We know that we can be difficult to live with but we do the best we can. We don't stop wanting to have close relationships but may need some time alone to rest at times. We are going to have days when we collapse with a flare. Losing the people we care about is very painful and one more type of grief that we may go through and can make us very sensitive to rejection. My hope is that this book may prevent some of that.

Even family members and friends that stick by us may have times that they get upset with us because they have unrealistic expectations. They may expect us to act normal or be the way we used to be. They may not want to hear about how we are really feeling or the problems we are having. Sometimes, they may want to try to "fix" what is wrong with us and they can't, leaving them feeling frustrated. It leaves us feeling frustrated too.

Sometimes the grief and depression causes us to avoid others and isolate ourselves. We often don't want to invite you to our home because we cannot keep it clean and neat the way we want it to be. We may feel guilty that we can't do what we think we should be doing. It may be a real effort for us to reach out to others, even those we love and care about. If you don't hear from us, please contact us and see how we are doing.

Other Symptoms and Associated Conditions

We have talked about pain and pressure but we probably also have stiffness, especially in the morning and after sitting still. We can have numbness and tingling. We have a reduced tolerance for exercise and muscle pain with exercise. We can have muscle twitching. Some of us also have myofascial pain, where we have tight bands of muscle and connective tissue that are painful. This is different than fibromyalgia pain and is treated differently. A lot of us also have arthritis so our joints may hurt in addition to our muscles.

Headaches, especially migraines, are common in those with fibromyalgia. We can be sensitive to odors, bright lights, noise, medications, certain foods and temperature (especially cold). Changes in weather can affect us. Some of us have ringing in our ears or pain in the temporo-mandibular joint (TMJ). Our coordination can be impaired and almost half of us have problems with balance. We seem to be more prone to allergies.

In addition to light sleep where we awaken easily, we are more likely to have restless leg syndrome or grinding of our teeth. We may have insomnia where we have difficulty falling asleep even when tired or get a falling sensation as we start to drift off that wakes us up. Some of us also have sleep apnea.

Many of us have irritable bowel syndrome with abdominal cramping, bloating and diarrhea and/or constipation. We can also have irritable bladder so that we need to urinate more frequently.

I suspect that a lot of these are a result of overactive nerves, just as the pain is a result of the nerves being overly sensitive to painful stimuli. We are more likely to become anxious for the same reason. I wouldn't be surprised if eventually treatment of fibromyalgia becomes something that neurologists handle rather than rheumatologists.

It is not unusual for people with fibromyalgia to gain weight as a result of not being able to do as much. It is hard to exercise when you are in pain and exercise might make it worse. We may also opt to eat fast or easy-to-fix foods because we don't have the energy to cook. As a result of poor diet, less exercise and weight gain, we may develop type 2 diabetes.

I'm sure by now you have gotten the picture that this is not an easy condition to live with. Despite all of our health issues, we try to make the best of things and do what we can. In the next sections, I will take you through a typical day to help you get a better sense of what life with fibromyalgia is like and then I will try to give you ways you can help us (and things that are not helpful).

A Day in the Life

I try to make sure that I get eight hours of sleep at night so if I have to get up early to go somewhere, I go to bed early. Whenever I get up, I usually take my time and stretch before getting out of bed because I am normally stiff and sore.

After a trip to the bathroom, my first priority is to put some coffee on and do some exercise. Both of these help me feel more awake and alert and give me some energy to get going. I usually (actually more like consistently) do not feel like exercising and have to push myself to do it because I know that, in the long run, I will feel better. If I have to go out, I will clean up and get ready to go and have breakfast if there is time. Otherwise, I will grab a piece of cheese to take with me along with more coffee.

If I don't have to go anywhere, I will have some quiet time to meditate and write in my journal. I usually wait to have breakfast so that I have the energy to cook something and then do something quiet, like reading emails, until I feel like getting cleaned up and dressed. If it is a day when I have very little energy, I may not get dressed and save the energy to work on my writing. If I'm flaring and/or having difficulty concentrating on my writing, I may read a book (light fiction, not anything that takes a lot of focus). I read a lot of books.

Meals are a big part of what I use my energy for because it is important to me to eat healthy food. This means I don't want to eat processed food and so I have to make the effort to prepare meals and clean up afterward. I also have to shop at least once a week for groceries. I make an effort to fix foods made from scratch but sometimes don't feel up to fixing what I planned and go for something easier. I buy some vegetables already cut up, even though it costs more because it is easier. Most of our meals are pretty simple. It is just too much work to do things like baking or making complicated recipes. I often use paper plates to cut down on dishes and try to use as few pans as possible and even so, I may soak them rather than washing them immediately. By the time I cook the meal, I'm ready to rest.

What we experience isn't the kind of tired you get from physical exertion but rather an overall fatigue that is hard to explain. It is mental as well as physical. I have to really push myself to do even simple things like making phone calls. Everything is an effort. Between forgetting to do things and having to push myself to get anything done, I have a lot of days when not much does get done. My mind has all kinds of great ideas about what I would like to do but I just can't get myself to do them. It is not like depression because I am a fairly positive, upbeat person. I don't feel sad; I just feel chronically exhausted and achy.

I like to play dulcimer and guitar with two groups on weekends. Every week, I tell myself that I'm going to practice between sessions. This is something I enjoy but I rarely do. Just getting the dulcimer or guitar and music out is an effort and I also forget that this is something I want to do unless I schedule it. I have a calendar that I write things on so I won't forget and sometimes forget to look at it. I feel disorganized. This week, I didn't go to the Sunday afternoon group and chose to pick berries instead. I also didn't feel up to going out on Wednesday and didn't go to either of the activities I could have gone to.

One thing I do every day is to "chat" with my friends in my on-line support group. Because they understand, they are my closest friends. This is a place where I can share my joys and my frustrations. I also spend a lot of time with on-line activities such as learning things through webinars, seeing what my family and friends are up to on facebook, plus researching, writing and looking for ways to promote my books.

I spent several hours at the Laundromat this week doing the laundry and on another day, I did the grocery shopping plus ran a few other errands. I only left the house on three out of seven days. In a typical week, I go out about four days a week for about three or four hours at a time. Some days I need to go out because of volunteer activities. These are usually scheduled so I will almost always force myself to go do these things where I am more likely to skip things that are optional. This is especially true for things that occur later in the day by which time I may not have a lot of energy left. When I haven't made a firm commitment to be somewhere, it is easy to give in to the fatigue.

How You Can Support Us

One of the most important things you can do is to believe us. We really do have a real condition that causes real pain, a lack of energy and a bunch of other symptoms. It is insulting to tell us that it is "all in our heads" like we are imagining it. Believe me, we have heard this far too often and we really don't want to hear it again. It isn't psychological. It is possible that we might have some mental health issues in addition to the fibromyalgia, just like anyone else might have but the fibromyalgia is not a result of mental illness. If we seem to be having problems, support us in getting help. Do not try to diagnose us or tell us what to do. Leave this to the appropriate professionals. Acknowledge that we are suffering and ask what you can do to help us.

Continue to include us in social activities. Yes, we might cancel but we really do want to spend time with the people we care about and appreciate invitations even if we can't go. We like to have fun just as much as anyone else and love to get out and do things. We want to do as much as we can, especially enjoyable things like being with our family and friends. Encourage us to have fun, even while you recognize that we might not be able to do as much as we used to do. Don't get angry if we can't go or go but then ask to leave an activity early. We are not doing this to annoy you; we are doing it to take care of ourselves.

Allow us to decide how much we are capable of doing and don't tell us to push through the pain and keep going. We have to listen to our bodies because we are the ones who will suffer the consequences if we do too much. We have all pushed ourselves too hard and know what happens when we do this. Sometimes it is worth it but it is better if we can avoid throwing ourselves into a flare. One day of pushing too hard has the potential to result in a week long flare. If we say we need to rest, support our need to do that.

Recognize that our pain is real, even if you don't understand it. Don't try to compare whatever pain you might have with ours. What you can do while having your pain and what I can do while having my pain is like comparing apples and oranges. We are all different. It is not a competition. Pain is a subjective experience that can be affected by many factors. Even if you can't see a reason for our pain, we still feel it. We have learned to hide it and to live with it but it still affects us.

Accept us as we are. When someone you care about has something wrong, it is natural to want to fix it. You can't fix us but you can listen to us and try to understand us. If you want to tell us about the wonderful drug that your Aunt Dorothy is taking, that is fine but don't expect us to get too excited. We have been disappointed by enough miracle drugs in the past. If you tell us about someone who has been cured of fibromyalgia, expect us to be skeptical. At this time, there is no cure. Anyone who says they are "cured", didn't have fibromyalgia in the first place. They just had something with some similar symptoms or they are saying this to try to get us to buy their product. We and our friends who have this condition keep an eye on the research in case there is some amazing discovery but we aren't holding our breath. The latest theory I have read indicates that it could be virus induced but I will wait for the research study to be completed and replicated before I believe this. We do like to hear about things that could help us feel better, especially if people we know have tried them and gotten good results.

Be realistic in your expectations. We are not the same as we used to be before we got this condition. We not only have the symptoms to deal with but also have to deal with fall-out like struggling to hold on to our jobs or trying to cope after losing our jobs. We don't need the pressure of trying to be someone we can't be anymore. We do the best we can so please accept that and don't get upset with us. Recognize that we may need to have some quiet time alone from time to time but that we still want you to be part of our lives.

Encourage us. We are often going through some tough times and it helps to have our family and friends there to support us. If you see that we are struggling and you are able to help, please do. We may not know how to ask for help. Sometimes, just being there for us can mean a lot to us.

Bring us joy. Tell us jokes, take us to see funny movies, make us laugh and do things with us that we enjoy. That will help us get our minds off the pain and the things we can't do. Encourage us with our dreams of what we might be able to do. Help us to see the positives and possibilities in life. Give us things to look forward to. Having a positive attitude helps with the pain so anything you can do to foster this is a good thing. We really need to have positive people around us so that we can stay positive. Help us to see things that we can be grateful for by looking for things in your own life that you are grateful for and sharing them.

Encourage us to join a support group, either locally or online. Much as we love our families and friends, we need to be able to vent to others who are going through the same problems that we are. Support group members are also a great source of information since people who have had fibromyalgia for a long time probably understand it better than your average doctor. They certainly know more about what life with fibromyalgia is like on a day to day basis and can suggest things that help.

Be open-minded and willing to learn. Reading this book is an excellent first step. The person you care about can tell you more about what they are experiencing if you are willing to listen. Since each of us is unique and may have some different symptoms, this is important. We also are going to be affected differently on different days. What was easy yesterday, might be hard today and vice versa. While this disease is not supposed to be progressive (according to the medical literature), we frequently get worse over time. In fact, everyone I know who has it has seen this happen, despite our efforts to maintain our health. A part of this is getting older and developing other conditions but we are also seeing the fibromyalgia getting worse. We are constantly having to adjust to this and you will have to also. Don't give up on us. Continue to love and support us. Share what you have learned here and stand up for us.

I hope that this book has helped you to understand more about what those of us with fibromyalgia are going through. If it has given you some insight into this syndrome and what you can do to help us, please leave a positive review on Amazon (at the bottom of the sales page).

If you have further questions, you can reach me through my facebook page:

(http://www.facebook.com/JanetLBlackpeacefulheartpress)

or my webpage:

(http://ecochristian.wix.com/peaceful-heart-press).

On behalf of all those who suffer from fibromyalgia, thank you for caring about us.

Printed in Great Britain
by Amazon